How to Start a Biotech Company

Sourish Saha, PhD
Samantha Holvey, EMHL
Anandhi Narasimhan, MD
Anales Debhaumik, PhD
Manisha Brahmachary, PhD
Mayukh Samanta, PhD

Table of Contents

Background
In 1919, Karl Ereky, a Hungarian Engineer coined the term "Biotechnology" which describes the use of human technology based on using biology to turn raw materials into socially active products. Almost a century later the vision of Ereky is impacting a large number of companies and research institutions.

Modern biotechnology has its roots in the 1970s in Northern California and has now become a worldwide industry which produces various medicines for patients. It now boosts of sectors such as healthcare (biologics, devices, diagnostics) agriculture (genetically modified organism, food safety), industry and environment (biofuels, biomaterials, pollution) and biodefense (vaccines, biosensors). This book will be primarily on healthcare.

Drug is a medicinal substance for prevention management or cure of an illness. FDA which stands for the United States Food and Drug Administration must give approval of all drugs before they are sold to the general public. Likewise most countries have such regulatory bodies that evaluates drugs following global guidelines before it is given for public consumption. Most common amongst drugs are the synthesized drugs like Aspirin, the Pharmaceutical industry manufactures synthetic drugs, whilst the biotechnological has given birth to a newer class of drugs: The Biologic.

Biologics are drugs from living organism and consists of curative proteins such as, DNA vaccines, monoclonal antibodies and peptibodies. This in essence is a combination of the active portion of a protein (peptide) with a portion of the inherent structure of an antibody as well as experimental modalities like gene therapy, stem cell therapy, antisense nucleotides and RNA viruses. A host of biotechnology drugs are Proteins derived from amino acids. These proteins are the driving force and perform all functions within a cell. As cells produce proteins naturally, the biotechnological companies use chemicals but make utilization of cells to produce biologics.

Note: [To market a new drug from discovery to its ultimate sale takes about 10 years to 15 years and cost upwards of $ 1 billion. One in ten new research drugs become successful and companies therefore depend on the revenue of a successful drug to offset the cost incurred for the failure of the other research drugs.]

The Science
The biotechnology industry is fully dependent on living organisms. The cell being the basic unit, living organism consists of one or multiple cells and some organisms are unicellular like bacteria and yeast. Humans are multi cellular having trillions of cells. All cells have a common mode of survival, and Biotechnology combines these modalities to manufacture drug to treat diseases and improve health. In order to comprehend the cell process specific input in detailed functioning of the cell is required.

- Cells Reproduce (mitosis): Before it divides, a cell makes a copy of the DNA and the other cell parts. From the original cell it forms two identical cells and these are referred to as the daughter cells. These cells then grow to their intended size.

- Cells Metabolize: This is a process by which cells maintains a living state by harnessing nutrients, break down into large and small molecules, produce energy by building molecular blocks, which in turn are used to create new cell structures and control cellular function.

- Cells Respond to stimuli: Unicellular and multicellular organisms respond to a whole range of stimuli both internal and external. For instance plants grow towards the source of light for photosynthesis and in order to produce energy. This response is essential for its survival. Cells can also adapt since organism may thrive or die according to their adaptability in adverse environmental conditions like, change in temperature, solute concentration, oxygen supply and exposure to hazardous agents.

Parts of an Animal Cell

This can be divided into three broad sections like the cell membrane, the cytoplasm (includes organelles) and the nucleus.

Nucleus: Contains most of the DNA and functions as the control center of the cell. It is encompassed by a membrane that releases molecules in and out of the nucleus in order to safeguard the DNA. The DNA does not ever leave the nucleus.

Cell Membrane:

The surrounding border of a cell is the cell membrane which controls the inflow and outflow of the cell. Inside the cell membrane are receptors which act as storage facility for molecules. When a specific type of molecules enters a receptor, chemical reaction takes place which in turn creates a cellular response. Blockage in a receptor evokes no response since signaling is not present. This is how biologic therapy works. They attach to receptors and interrupt the cell signaling process or others by invoking the signaling molecule.

Organelles:

There are various types of organelles inside the cytoplasm of a cell performing multiple of functions. Ribosomes makes protein, Mitochondria produces energy. By a mechanism of folding endoplasmic reticulum and transport specific proteins, golgi bodies help to modify proteins for transportation within the cell. Vacuoles store cellular wastage for disposal.

Within one minute Ribosomes can assemble an average size protein.

DNA

All cells contain deoxyribonucleic acid or DNA and thereby it is the foremost factor in cell construction and operation. It (DNA) is constructed in sections called Chromosomes within which are specific parts of DNA called genes. Genes vary in length, and stores information that a cell needs to manufacture proteins which in turn impacts cellular functions.

Note: [In animal cells, Mitochondria are the only organelles to have their own DNA. Mutations or divisions in Mitochondria DNA leads to diseases like Kearns-Sayre syndrome causing loss of heart, eye and muscle movement functions]

The DNA consist of four basic "Building Blocks" called nucleotides and is a code storing information. The length of DNA is very long, and the order of the nucleotides dictates the information stored. Three distinct components constitute the nucleotide namely a deoxyribose, sugar, a phosphate group and a base. There are four types of bases: adenine (A), thymine (T), guanine (G) and cytosine (C). The basic sequence of As, Ts, Cs, and Gs in DNA imparts meaning to the cell, similar to alphabets in a word imparts meaning to it, or even in a story in which the word appears. The diverse nature of organisms is a result of an unlimited combination of bases- As, Ts, Gs and Cs. Although every organism contains DNA but, the arrangement and number of bases vary for each organism.

DNA is referred to as double helix because two strands of nucleotides bond together in a very exact manner. For instance, As bond within Ts, Cs bond with Gs, resulting in A.T and C-G combinations. These are called base pairs. In every human cell, the length of DNA is equivalent to 3 billion base pairs. If the structure of DNA is flattened, it would resemble a ladder with two side rails (phosphate and ribose groups) and rungs (base pairs) between them. This enables DNA to be very stable and store vast amounts of information.

Humans have 23+ 23=46 pairs of chromosomes, half from each parent, and Chromosomal abnormalities can be numeric or structural

Most cells in an organism contains the exact same DNA, but not all genes are always active or turned on, but whenever a gene is turned on, the encoded information helps to produce or express, the enclosed protein. When not active or turned on it cannot express proteins. Therefore, depending on the need of the cell function, genes become active or inactive. Many diseases are a result of this impropriety.

Mutations:

—

A change in the DNA sequence is called mutation and is basically a result of environmental factors like exposure to radiation or chemical toxins. Mutations can also be a result of natural process of DNA replication, wherein a cell is copying 3 billion base pairs in 20 hours. Bases can be substituted, deleted or repeated and this change in DNA sequence may cause in harboring dysfunctional proteins or just the opposite. Accumulation of mutation over a period of time in genes can result in differences in species.

Genomes:

This is a term which refers to all genetic information in an organism. The human genome is the entire DNA content found in a human. Genomes are made up of the same bases: As, Ts, Gs and Cs. The difference lies in the sequence and numbers of base pairs and genes. The numbers of base pairs do not correspond to the number of genes and hence the two are independent of each other. Human genome has 3 billion base pairs and approximately 20,000 to 25,000 codes for genes. Only 3 percent of human genome codes for genes, 97 percent are noncoding DNA or in other words do not have instructions for creating proteins. Biologists are yet to discover this strange phenomenon but concur that it may be due to evolution in species or regulatory functions within the cell.

Note: [Variation in individual nucleotides occur at the rate of one in every 13,000 base pairs in most organisms. In humans it is one in every 1200. However, most of these mutations do not adversely affect us and only a few causes dysfunctional protein or diseases status]

It is to be noted that the number of base pairs and genes have no relevance to the intelligence or physical capability of an organism. An amoeba genome is a unicellular organism which has 670 billion base pairs compared to 3 billion in a human genome. Yet the human is more complex, intelligent and physically capable organism.

Proteins:

These are along chains of amino acids that fold into intricate and complex 3-D shapes. In a gene the DNA sequences determines the order of amino acids and their sequence determines the shape and functions of the protein. The highest number of genes in an organism is 60,000 for the bacteria that causes trichomoniasis, three times as many as in a human genome.

Transcription and Translation are two complicated and multiple steps in protein synthesis.

Transcription:

During this process the original DNA code is rewritten into a molecule called messenger RNA (mRNA). mRNA consists of nucleotides that are slightly different from DNA nucleotides. RNA molecules are similar to DNA but contain ribose sugar of single strand and use all U or uracil, in place of T, or thymine as one of the four possible bases.

Translation:

During translation ribosomes help to assemble individual amino acids into proteins and also bind to mRNA. Three mRNA nucleotides constitute a Codon which is the code for an amino acid. In the process of translation, transfer RNA (tRNA) decodes mRNA and attaches to the corresponding amino acid. Therefore, a specific combination of amino acids are linked together as required by the sequence of nucleotides on the mRNA.

Short chains of amino acids are called peptides and the long one is polypeptide which fold into a functional protein. Numerous types of protein perform various functions within and between cells. Proteins called enzymes bind or break molecules. Signaling molecule transmit messages from one to another, as also protein receptors which receive signals through a communication channel known as Signal Transduction. Some proteins move substances out of a cell whilst structural proteins impart shape to cells and organism. Proteins are involved in cellular recognition and identification, while others such as antibodies help in defense of organism against diseases.

How Biology Drives Biotechnology

Biology is a study of life and the basic unit of life is the cell. Biotechnology, which is based on biology, studies the structure and the function of cells and uses this information to develop products. Researchers use their knowledge of genes, proteins and cell parts to determine the difference between diseased and healthy cells. They use their expertise on how to affect alterations in diseased cells, and then create unique medical diagnostics, devices and therapies.

Understanding Diseases Mechanisms:

Drug research and development (R&D) begins with an intensive study of underlying biology of specific diseases. Biotechnology produces medicines to treat a particular disease process. To design and develop new drugs, researchers must delve into the disease process involved. Certain pertinent queries in this respect are: How does a person get afflicted by the disease? Which particular cells become affected? Is this disease genetic? Is the cell turned off or on? Which proteins are being produced or not as compared to healthy cells? Whether the disease is caused by a Pathogen and what is the interaction between the pathogen and the involved person?

Note: [Biotechnology is one of the most R&D intensive industry in the world and the United States is the undisputed world leader]

In the early stage of drug development, it is necessary to collate information on disease mechanism. Proper understanding of fundamental biology lead to effective therapies for the patients. Consider for instance autoimmune disorder. This disease symptoms occur when a person's immune system reacts to attack proteins, tissues in the body leading to inflammation. Researchers concur that tumor necrosis factor (TNF) has a major role in regulating inflammation. That there is a surfeit of TNF production in diseases like rheumatoid arthritis, psoriasis, psoriatic arthritis, juvenile idiopathic arthritis, and ankylosing spondylitis. Excessive production of TNF is harmful to joints, skin, and other parts of the body. Biotechnology has helped to develop medicines to inhibit the activity of TNF.

Models for Studying Diseases:

One method is to collect samples of diseased cells and healthy cells and grow them using a method called Cell Culture. In this process the cells are incubated and fed with specialized growth media, whereby they divide and express genes in order to produce proteins. By observing this interaction between healthy and diseased cells, it is possible to comprehend the disease mechanism.

Another divergent approach is to study shared or similar genes and protein equivalents in other species. Since all the cells in organisms perform similar functions, genes and proteins found in humans are also found in other organisms. Function of human genes have been discovered by studying parallel genes in non-humans. It is due to this fact that we have understood how specific genes, and proteins direct the function of human cells-both healthy and diseased.

Note: [Computational biology involves computer science, applied mathematics and statistics]

Bioinformatics:

This is a combination of biology, computer science and information technology into one set format. The basic principle of bioinformatics is to understand and develop biology. It throws the gauntlet to computer programmers to design innovative databases, so as to permit easy access to existing and new data. Volumes of scientific data is generated on a daily basis. Companies have analyzed and computed this data to study cell activity, and develop diagnostic tools, therapies and preventive medicines. Bioinformatics has become a boon for advance in Biotechnology and helps to focus on nucleotide sequences, genes and amino acid chains.

Biomarkers

These are markers or substances that help to evaluate, and also measure normal biological processes, pertaining to disease conditions, treatment and intervention, Biomarkers reflect physiological indicators like blood pressure or heart rate. However, now molecule biomarkers are being used to evaluate prostate specific Antigens (PSA). Elevated levels of PSA can indicate prostate cancer.

Note: [Comparative studies are being conducted in respect of genome structure and function in various species. Genomic sequences have helped to detect bacteria causing ESCHERICHIA COLI (E.coli), the yeast SACCHAROMYCES CEREVISIAE, round worm CAENORHABDITIS ELEGANS, the fruit fly DROSOPHILA MELANOGASTER etc. Comparative studies using laboratory mouse and human genome are being conducted]

If the biomarker test indicates a positive strain, it can help to diagnose a disease and determine the treatment process. It also indicates prognosis i.e. how the disease will progress if not treated. This is a quantum leap in R&D for development of newer biotechnological diagnostic tools.

Note: [Genetic biomarkers are tests that study DNA fragments to ascertain the cause of disease or susceptibility to certain genetic disorders]

Research has indicated modification and changes in cellular activity, such as protein synthesis in multiple of diseases, conditions. Biomarkers help to specify disease progression and can be used as, a development tool for testing and drug discovery. A study in animal modules with Biomarkers can help to deduce effectiveness. In disease management. It indicates whether a drug is effective and at what dosage. Dose requirements may vary in patients as well as response to a specific drug.

Proteomics:

A chain of proteins in an organism is called proteome. A study of this involves protein structure and function. Proteins control cellular function as a whole. It can help to indicate in any specific cell of an organism time, hormonal changes and stress. Proteomics research can specify all proteins involved in protein synthesis and protein folding in their exact 3-D shape. For effective functioning any small alterations or structural defects may result in protein disease.

Note: [More than 200 therapeutics and vaccines have been discovered by biotechnology including medicines for cancer, diabetes and autoimmune disorders like HIV/AIDS. Most of these products are therapeutic proteins.]

To understand the structure, function and interaction of proteins within cells is a facet of drug discovery. Proteins are responsible for normal or abnormal functioning which may result in a disease. The molecule named drug target brings about the necessary changes by hitting its target.

Cancer: From Biology to Treatment:

Bio-informatics is a pioneer in cancer research. It helps to analyze proteins and develop new remedies that influences specific cellular processes. Cancer biology explores all avenues of a cancer cell. The molecular basis determines methods to develop diagnostics and treatment. Cancer start with changes in one cell or multiple cells which reproduce in an uncontrolled manner. In healthy cells, division and growth are regulated. But cancer cells continuously divide creating an opportunity for mutations, which may be a result of environment or DNA replication. As the cell replicate and grow a mass (tumor) is formed, the cell breaks away from tumor to metastasize and spread in the bloodstream, or the lymphatic system of the body to create more tumors.

Cancer can be treated with surgery, radiation and chemotherapy. Biotechnology has brought about significant hormone therapies, biologics and targeted therapies such as monoclonal antibodies.

Technology

Technology has brought about a plethora of changes in the evolution of laboratory techniques, tools and a focus on platform technologies. To understand these changes, it is necessary to gather basic knowledge about what goes on in the laboratory.

Restriction Enzymes:

A process of biotechnology is called genetic engineering, which is a combination of DNA sequences producing recombinant proteins as eventual therapeutics. This process utilizes restriction enzymes (endonucleases) in bacteria. These enzymes cut viral DNA into small nonfunctional pieces, thus protecting the bacterium from any invading virus.

There are hundreds of restriction enzymes, each recognizing a specific DNA called a restriction site. EcoR1, a restriction enzyme found in E. coli identifies and cuts at the six-base sequence GAATTS. HaeIII, a restriction enzyme found in Haemophilus-aegyptius, identifies and cuts at the four base sequence GGCC.

Note: [More than 3,800 restriction enzymes have been identified by scientists and 600 are commercially available in the marketplace.]

Irrespective of its origin DNA is made up of the same four bases i.e. As, Ts, Gs. and Cs. HaeIII detects any DNA segment and cuts it every time it encounters sequence GGCC. The key characteristics of restriction enzymes are that it is specific and reproducible. This helps scientists to utilize restriction enzymes for manipulating DNA.

The opposite of cutting is pasting. The sealing of two DNA segments is achieved by DNA ligase a protein enzyme by a process called ligation. This ability to cut and paste DNA is the premise on which genetic engineering is based.

Note: [Recombinant DNA technology and the discovery of restriction endonucleases earned the noble prize of 1978 to scientists Daniel Nathans, Werner Arber and Hamilton Smith.]

Recombinant DNA

When segments of DNA are cut and pasted together whereby a new DNA called recombinant DNA emerges, and this can be introduced into cells to produce new cells. These cells possess new characteristics, and this genetic alteration can include a single-base letter change or multiple gene changes. The change in a host cell is done by a VECTOR, which physically carry the DNA. A host cell can comprise of bacteria, yeast, plant, insect of mammalian.

Common bacterial vectors include plasmids and phages. A plasmid is s DNA of circular proportion which can engineer and carry a gene of interest. A phage is a genetically engineered virus that injects DNA into bacteria. Cells containing recombinant DNA, are usually referred to as genetically modified transgenic or transformed cells, the process is commonly known as transformation.

Note: [1982, human insulin was approved by FDA in the United States, and this is an instance of the first medicine via recombinant DNA technology]

Recombinant Proteins:

Recombinant DNA is used in the manufacturing of Recombinant Proteins. The host cell utilizes DNA information and its inherent cell machinery to produce the encoded protein. When these proteins are used as human therapeutics, the host cells must produce and grow in large proportion in order to meet demand. This protein (recombinant protein) is isolated, purified and verified for quality and activity before its marketability.

Producing a protein with proper chain of amino acids entails intense processing in order to be functional and be active. A significant number of human proteins are glycosylated, which signifies that a particular pattern of sugar molecules are linked to them. If translated and not glycosylated, then there is the possibility of its malfunctioning. Addition of phosphate group knows as phosphorylation allows the protein to become active. A wilder range of functions get enhanced by addition of other biochemical groups.

Recombinant Proteins include vaccines, hormones, monoclonal antibodies, and hematopoietic growth factors for treating patients of cancer, AIDS, allergies, asthma and a host of different conditions. Due to advanced technology in recent times the number of recombinant proteins has increased significantly.

Cell Culture:

Cell Culture is a technique of growing cells in controlled conditions in a laboratory. Transformed bacteria cells and transformed animal cells are processed in order to manufacture recombinant protein drugs. Simple proteins are produced involving DNA technology in bacterial cell cultures, more complex proteins that are glycosylated are formulated in animal cell cultures.

In the process of cell culture, cells are grown in petri dishes or flasks that contain liquid media. This provides nutrients for cell growth, and the cultures are grown in an incubator which maintains proper temperature and environment. Gas mixtures of oxygen and carbon dioxide are often required. The maintenance of specific conditions is a must as any variation will have negative impact in the product produced. Commercial production of proteins has to be sufficient to meet demand. Since there are limitations in growing cells in petri dishes or flasks, it is commercially more viable to transfer cell cultures to larger vessels called bioreactors. Biotechnology scientists have the facility of various state-of-art laboratory equipment in their quest to further the cause of genetic engineering.

Thermocycler:

Thermocycler is a machine that replicates DNA which results in Polymerase chain reaction (PCR). PCR is a series of cycles utilizing a minimal amount of original DNA in order to copy and amplify it. Each three-step cycle doubles the amount of DNA present and is like a photocopier for DNA. A single piece can churn out million copies of the same DNA. PCR enables scientists with sufficient DNA for their laboratory work. There are various applications for PCR including DNA sequence production, gene for use in creating recombinant proteins.

Note: [For invention and development of Polymerase chain reaction, the noble prize in chemistry was given to Kary Banks Mullis in 1983.]

Gel Electrophoresis:

For analyzing DNA fragments gel electrophoresis is commonly used. This technical apparatus helps in separating DNA fragments within a gel by allowing electricity to run through it. The fragment is negatively charged and thereby shift to the positive pole of the gel apparatus. The larger DNA fragments move slowly than the smaller ones as they receive resistance from the matrix gel.

There are various types of electrophoresis and separation of gel being one type and types of molecules being the other. DNA, RNA and proteins can all be separated using this method with the relevant apparatus. It has many applications in both clinical and research labs and is generally applied for verification of PCR products. It can therefore be used to cross-check on whether the reaction emanates from the correct DNA fragment.

DNA Microarrays:

DNA microarrays is a gene chip which is a small piece of glass or silicon divided into thousands of sections in a grid pattern. Each section has a single-stranded gene fragment corresponding to either a healthy or diseased gene. An individual's DNA is separated into single strands and attached to a fluorescent dye and then washed over the microarray. The DNA binds to any complementary DNA on the slide and if the sequence is present it becomes a double stranded DNA. The use of computer helps to locate and measure spots on the double stranded fluorescent tagged DNA. Each DNA must match the gene fragment exactly and bind, to indicate the presence of a healthy or diseased DNA. Microarrays are a potent tool for analysis of genes. They are used in genetic testing and, for comparative study of genetic information of individual or species and discovery of drugs.

Researchers are using microarrays in identifying genes and with recombinant DNA technologies. Other microarrays include protein, tissue, chemical compounds and antibody. Thousands of data points are analyzed at a time.

Note: [Microarrays are capable of generating enormous data so that special storage facility is required. There are both public and private microarray data bases]

Drug Discovery

Scientists normally search for molecules of either chemical or biological agents that can alter a disease process. They strive to find ways to change one or several molecular or cellular processes that occur in the affected cells of a diseased tissue or organ.

Initiating Drug Research:

To identify unknown medical need and current treatment procedure is the first step in this direction. The expertise is also needed. Financial resources and regulatory considerations are taken into account as well.

Note: [According to the National center for Health in the United States, the top five diseases in 2005 were heart disease, cancer, stroke, chronic lower respiratory afflictions and diabetes.]

Target Discovery:

Identification of a medical necessity, and consideration of available financial resources, spurs scientists to examine closely the biology behind the disease. Since the human body is a very complex system, options are considered for intervening and earmarking the target. Target is a molecule and plays a crucial role in a disease. There are 8000 known therapeutic targets in existence. These can be secreted factors, cell surface receptors or can point to pathways within a cell. The principle aim is to develop a drug which interferes with the disease process and ensures tangible benefits as well as minimizing side effects.

The therapeutic approach is not the same for all targets as their response is varied and so it is necessary to differentiate between healthy and diseased cells. The molecule is the main factor in a disease and the causes are many. In a disease which is inherited it can be noted that, there is a difference in the expression and sequence of genes resulting in abnormal cell function. In some cases, the target can be in excess, deficient or absent. So, it becomes necessary to decide whether the target is to be blocked or enhanced or replaced for normal healthy function. Sometimes diseases are caused by external pathogen like virus or bacterium. The pathogen produces molecules thereby damaging host organism cells. Here the pathogen will display molecules in the individual so infected, contrary to that of a healthy person. The aim of target discovery is the detection of these different molecules by technology such as microarray, protein electrophoresis, Mass Spectrometry (MS), DNA sequencing and computerized imaging.

Since cell to cell interaction are very complex, the time taken in target discovery can span many years. There can be an involvement of multiple mechanisms and the points requiring intervention. The characteristics of a healthy or diseased cell can be very minute, complex and in some cases identification methods are yet to be invented.

Note: [The genetic and molecular basis of a disease is called the studying of disease mechanism.]

Target Validation:

After a target is identified it has to be validated. This comprises of two components, firstly to ascertain that the target molecule is responsible for the disease, and secondly to confirm the need for therapeutic intervention. The formulation of a safe and effective drug for human testing is considered and this process completes the second phase of target validation. Time, cost and technology are the prime concerns in target validation. At the basic level of this validation it is necessary to create the disease in a sample of healthy tissues and then block the target to restore healthy condition. This experiment is conducted in cell culture or animal models. The aim is to select the specific representative model which will work. Some people who are born without specific functional molecules express certain disease types. Samples derived from such individuals is another way of validating a target.

Target molecules includes receptors, enzymes, ion channels, growth factors, cytokines and DNA binding proteins. The common factor is the involvement of these targets in Signal Transduction processes within cells. Signal transduction pathways control cell division, differentiation, protein synthesis and programmed cell death (apoptosis). Cell culture is the initial phase of study and if found positive, then an animal model is used. Suitable animal model has to be created as it is not always easy to find one in an existing animal model or may not be similar to a human disease state. Sometimes a drug is specific to humans, unable to recognize the animal models target as the animal display immune response that negates any therapeutic effect. A disease in question is the Alzheimer's syndrome. Only recently has research been done in mouse models. A study also analyzes the various effects of preclinical symptoms within the cell culture and animal models. At times the target is expressed on those cells and tissues besides the others in the disease process. Questions generally asked relate to cells and tissues of a drug candidate having adverse effect on other cells and tissues, does it give an immune response, does it stimulate similar targets or generate toxicity?

This preclinical work helps to establish further human trials if the drug candidate shows promise. Even if the drug gets marketing approval, surveillance continues after administration to patients.

Note: [Nowadays, Scientists use computer simulation to portray drug target interactions and it acts as a guideline to drug discovery.]

Screening:

High-throughput screening is a combination process of robotics and data processing that quickly identifies the compounds, antibodies or genes that modulate a particular biomolecular pathway. Potential drugs are tested for binding or biological activity against target molecules. Once a diseased candidate gets verified, research labs develop a testing method called ASSAY in order to determine or measure pharmacological activity of hundred thousands of molecules.

The assay helps to measure the estimated potential of a molecule to block or simulate a target. The measurement can either be simply to know the potential of a drug candidate to kill cancer cells, or the complex measurement of inhibiting an enzyme involved in a disease. A complex assay gives out pertinent information but at a high cost and a long time schedule.

Molecules having positive therapeutic potential are called lead molecules as they are composed of drug like properties like solubility, permeability, and stability. Researchers can optimize a drug candidate's ability to fight disease by changing its molecular structure, by application of combinatorial chemistry for small molecules and protein engineering for the larger variety.

Drug Design:

The basis of this design is in understanding the genetic and molecular base of a disease, and the information so given in selection of a specific therapeutic target. Drugs are designed to interact with the target. Rational drug design help in developing drugs suitable for a specific target in a disease. It also acts as a factor in achieving improved therapeutic potency with less side effects.

Scientists depend on image technology such as X-ray crystallography and 3-D structural information for enhancement of drug design strategies. If the target is on the exterior surface of the cell membrane or is secreted, protein therapeutics like monoclonal antibodies or peptides can be used. If they are on the interior of the cell, then only drugs that can cross the cell membrane like small molecules are used. The ultimate shape of a drug whether as a pill, liquid injection or spray determine the design of a drug candidate.

Drug Development

The lengthy process of drug discovery does not complete the process of drug development. It comprises of safety, efficacy, formulation and manufacture of the drug. Preclinical Studies are safety testing experiments involving humans in chain of studies called Clinical Trials.

Preclinical Studies

These are tests performed in a controlled environment using cell cultures and animals as models. The idea is to predict what the body does to the drug candidate, by way of pharmacokinetics, or vice versa pharmacodynamics, and whether there is a potential health hazard and toxic side effects.

Pharmacokinetic testing supplies data in regard to drug absorption and transportation. It indicates the cells and organs affected, break up of enzymes, the time it takes to do so or how the metabolites are eliminated from the body. Pharmacodynamics on the other hand examine dose response, monitor biochemical and physiological changes such as enzyme activities, heart rate, blood pressure and body temperature of subjects undergoing tests. It answers important questions regarding the body's response to the drug and the attendant toxicity in respect of the cells and organs. It also addresses the potential of a drug and its metabolites to kill or damage those cells or organs, initiate reproductive issues, cause cancer as well as birth defects and sterility. Pharmacokinetics and pharmacodynamics form the core of preclinical studies. These studies are mandatory in all countries which follow proper regulatory guidelines. Information from these studies are vital to calculate safe dosage during clinical trials. Ethical concerns and spiraling costs are impeding researchers to consider reducing the number of animal models to a minimal proportion. The United States monitor the care in case of laboratory animals by its Animal Welfare Act, which specifies that any organization receiving federal funding for research must create an Institutional Animal Care and use Committee (IACUC).

Animal models determine the effectiveness and the safety of new drug candidates. The use of KNOCK-OUTMICE or KNOCK-INMICE are tools for target validation. Knock-out mice are genetically altered to remove mouse versions of human disease genes. These genes can be knocked in to create mouse models having disease, conditions like cancer, diabetes, Alzheimer's and Parkinson's. Candidate drugs can then be given to humans after a thorough check of adverse side effects.

The study of safety and toxicity are done using CELL LINES, which are engineered to express genes that are responsible for adverse reactions. The decline in the use of animals is due to the creation of cell lines, which helps to speed up drug development processes. If the preclinical trials are proven to be safe, then the organization involved in research can submit an Investigational New Drug (IND) to the appropriate authorities for approval of clinical trials in humans.

Clinical Trials:

Clinical trials in humans are designed to assess drug safety, proper dosage, adverse reactions and chronic toxicity. They are conducted under guidelines such as FDA's Current Good Clinical Practice (cGCP), which ensures the safety of human test subjects, and conforms to the U.S Code of Human Research Ethics. Clinical trials are conducted in three phases and tests a large number of humans in each phase. Success in each phase leads to the next or lack of success results in the trials being halted and the drug suspended.

Since the time taken to conduct clinical trials are very lengthy, often an independent contract research organization (CRO) undertakes such ventures. They liaise with the sponsor organization and also ensure that, the volunteers subjected to these trials accept the risks involved. Participation as study subjects is voluntary, however each one of them have to sign a document called informed consent. The informed consent can be withdrawn by them at any time.

Phase 1:

This phase represents the testing of a new drug in humans to ascertain the drug's safety, tolerability and safe dosage range. The testing group averages between 20 to 50 volunteers who are free from disease. However, when testing oncology therapeutics, patients having cancer are chosen as subjects because involving healthy patients would be too risky as the side effects of chemotherapeutic agents are very pronounced.

Phase 2:

In this phase a large group of volunteers (100 to 300) who are suffering from the disease for which the drug is intended participate. Normally the group is divided into two distinct pairs, one studying the dosage aspect and the other the efficacy of the drug. New investigational drugs during this phase have a high failure rate because of efficacy and safety issues.

Phase 3:

The set goal in this phase is to determine the effectiveness of the drug, and its comparison with placebos or therapies already available and marketed. Thousands of volunteers are tested over a long period of time, stretching to several years in order to confirm long term safety of the drug. The research company files a new drug or biologics application with the country's regulatory body. In the U.S, a company would file a New Drug Application (NDA) for a small molecule drug or a BIOLOGIC LICENSE APPLICATION (BLA) for a large molecule drug to the FDA. Similarly, in Europe it can be filed with European Medicines Agency known as EMEA. On getting approval from the regulatory body, the drug can be produced mass scale in a facility so approved and then marketed. In the U.S the need to confirm to FDA's current good Manufacturing Practice (CGMP) is mandatory to ensure purity and safety of the product. There is a acute shortage of study subjects in conducting clinical trials worldwide.

Concluding Phase:

In this phase the main objective is to determine and monitor the drug's safety and efficacy when consumed by millions of diseased patients. Sometimes acute adverse reactions are reported, since the trials have been conducted on a limited group of people. In such a scenario the company voluntarily withdraws the drug, or the regulatory body does it. Further trials may or may not reinstate the concerned drug. The phases in product development or product pipeline averages 10 to 15 years for its completion. One in a thousand potential drugs will finally get approved.

Manufacturing Process

The manufacturing process of biologics is a complex process of biologics as it involves proteins which are large molecules variable in structure and sensitive to environmental conditions. It is a four-step process: production of a master cell line, growth of cells producing proteins, isolation and purification of proteins from cells and then preparing the biologic for patients. The manufacturing process can consume years and cost hundreds of millions of dollars.

Using R&D Specifications:

Initial production during this phase is limited to small scale manufacturing. Usually an injection or infusion in respect of biotechnology medicine and its final formulation and physical form is produced. Going by the data generated large scale production is planned. The scale-up and manufacturing adheres to CGMP guidelines in respect of safety and purity.

Common Cell Lines:

A large number of biotechnology products are proteins produced by cells grown in a culture media. Chinese hamster ovary (CHO) cells, non-secreting (NOS) cells and E. coli are cell lines involved in production of biotherapeutics with emphasis on monoclonal antibodies. CHO and NSO cells help to synthesize proteins like human cells do. Since they can produce and grow forever, they are called immortal cell lines. These cell lines are generally regarded as safe (GRAS) for producing therapeutic proteins. NSO cells have an advantage to produce antibodies but do not secrete or make any of their own antibody protein. Other suitable cells can also be used but, the selection of such cell lines will depend on the expertise of the company's research team. Such selection will hinge on the properties of the cells and regulatory requirements.

Scale-Up-Process:

The scale-up of a cell culture is complex and time consuming. Several months can elapse before a product is obtained. Production of a biotech product is divided into two parts: upstream and downstream. Upstream processes constitute production of protein product by using cells like microbial, insect or mammalian in culture growth. Downstream processes help in recovery, purification, formulation and packaging of the product.

Upstream Phase:

This is a process where researchers create and engineer to formulate a protein product. Once the desired cell line is achieved it is cryopreserved i.e. frozen in a large number of vials to create a CELL BANK. It is then removed and thawed from the cell bank for cell culture in a flask containing a small amount of growth media as little as 5ml. The media is the provider of nutrients and the environment for the cell to survive.

Scale-Up is achieved by a gradual transfer of growing cells into larger containers having larger media volumes, and these are constantly dividing due to favorable growth environment. More cells are present with each step and hence more protein product is generated.

Scale-up Monitoring:

This sets the stage for quicker growth of cells and thereby production of substantial protein product. Assays or other testing methods are used by scientists to measure CELL VIABILITY and concentration, product concentration and activity at each scale up stage for better monitoring.

Advanced laboratory environment helps to control physical environment for cell to grow. This is done manually in the nascent steps and helps to optimize growth parameters like temperatures, PH, nutrient concentration and oxygen level. Since this is a large and automated culture it can be grown in bioreactors. FERMENTATION and manufacturing stages helps technicians to monitor contamination, bacteria, yeast or other microorganisms. Contamination ruins an entire batch and so technicians maintain ASEPTIC conditions during this phase.

Quality Control and Quality Assurance:

These departments quality control (QC) and quality assurance (QA) are responsible to monitor scale-up activities, leading to manufacture and product development. QC department maintains product standards by assuring product quality during development and marketing stages. Quality assurance determine quality objectives.

Downstream Phase:

Isolation of the protein product from the cells is one of the major objectives of this phase. INTRACELLULAR PROTEINS found in the cells require special techniques for extraction and purification. The cell is burst open so that it releases the protein product for purification and isolates it from various components of the cell. Proteins which are extracted away from the cells (EXTRACELLULAR PROTEINS) are easier to isolate.

CLARIFICATION is the next step after harvesting the protein product. Here proteins are separated from cellular debris. A protein solution is applied to a series of chromatography columns and hence a pure protein product is derived. The process of COLUMN CHROMATOGRAPHY that separates proteins is dependent on physical and chemical properties like size, shape or change i.e. + or - . Further purification helps in removing residual DNA, and deactivates any viral particles.

Confirmed testing protocols help to verify the process of isolation and purification. The protein product thus obtained as per R&D specification is then packaged for use by physicians and patients.

Biotechnology Medicine

Advancement of technology in the sphere of application in cellular and molecular biology has created many wonderful products to treat or prevent diseases. Numerous products that include therapeutic proteins, monoclonal antibodies, vaccines, allergy immunotherapy drugs and also blood components and tissues and cells for transportation.

Therapeutic Proteins:

These are often referred to as biologics and makes use of recombination DNA technology. These biologics play a significant role in oncology, rheumatology, immunology, endocrinology and virology. Some of these biologics are now considered standard therapy and have been in use for more than 20 years. Others are in research and clinical trials.

Doctors have frequently used therapeutic proteins to replace or supplement natural body proteins, if found diminished in levels or lost due to the disease that the patient is suffering from. Most recombinant proteins are versions of natural body proteins, while others although not exact versions produce the same effect.

Vaccines:

These stimulate the immune system by providing protection in a particular disease. Initially, vaccines were made from inactivated or weakened virus unable to reproduce in the body, but capable to provide immunity if exposed to the live virus. Genetic engineering creates recombinant vaccines by inserting genes for desired antigens into a vector. The vector vaccine or carrier is basically a weakened virus or bacterium into which is inserted harmless genetic material from a specific disease causing organism. White blood cells in the body recognizes and attacks any foreign antigens. Recombinant vaccines do not cause any disease but have the antigen to mislead the body into a state of being attacked by a pathogenic virus. However, these vaccines are safe and easily grown and stored.

Antibodies:

The main focus of biologics centers around the production of fully human antibodies. These can attach to antigens found in pathogen and helps to destroy the same pathogen by the immune system. Antibodies can also attach to proteins on immune cells involved in auto immune responses, in diseased conditions like rheumatoid arthritis and multiple sclerosis. humanized antibodies are engineered to avoid rejection and are derived from human cells or human antibody genes.

Peptibodies:

These are therapeutic fusion proteins having qualities of both peptides and antibodies, having distinctive features and bind to human targets.

Diagnostics:

Recombinant DNA technology produces diagnostic tests for diseases like hepatitis and AIDS. Recombinant protein antigens act as reagents in enzyme-linked immunosorbent assay (ELISAs) for detection of Severe Acute Respiratory Syndrome (SARS).

Future of Biotechnology in Healthcare

Biotechnology offers more and better healthcare options, novel diagnostics and therapies for prevention and treatment of diseases. Although at an initial stage, it is ushering in an era of innovative medicines, diagnostics and technologies in development that hold great promise to better patients' lives.

Personalized Medicine:

This is a concept of treatment with therapy and medicine based on each patients' unique genetics make up for obtaining optimal results. Current medical practice is based on the average response across large group of people. Personalized Medicine is a new phenomenon whereby an individual patient's characteristics like age, gender, height, weight, diet and genetics environment are under consideration. This has led to the development of genomic personalized medicine which translates to medical care based on a patient's genotype or gene expression profile.

Pharmacogenomics:

This process in healthcare takes into account the individual's unique genomes which represent their genetic make-up. These genomes are likely to react differently to a specific drug and dose quantity. The task is to differentiate the drug and dose in individuals or groups who possess similar genetics. This process aids the physician in selecting and prescribing specific drugs, with dose levels that enable to combat a particular disease.

Rapid advances in DNA technology is the basis for both pharmacogenomics and personalized medicine. It helps in the determination of an individual's unique genetic make-up, and its difference with others. Variations in genomes as well as encoded proteins among individuals, have helped researchers to develop medicines specific to each patient. Pharmacogenomics and personalized medicine have made rapid strides in the sphere of clinical trials in drugs, screening technology resulting in enhanced healthcare and significant advances in preventive medicine.

Genetic Testing:

The discovery of single nucleotide polymorphism (SNPS) which is a single nucleotide change in the DNA sequence has revolutionized genetic testing. One of the common forms of genetic variation in individuals is called SNPs or "Snips". When a SNP occurs in a gene sequence that encodes a specific protein, it can alter that protein causing disease or susceptibility to a disease. Using technology to detect SNPs helps to accurately diagnose genetic diseases and facilitates that treatment process. Genetic testing presents a clear overview of risks associated with a disease and its possible prevention. More than 10 million SNPS have been identified in the human genome.

Gene Therapy:

This is a new area of applied genetics that uses recombinant DNA technology. Gene therapy involves inserting genes created by recombinant DNA technology into the cells and tissues of patients to treat the diseases. A study of inherited human disease involving defective genes are now being done, in order to replace them with functional genes. Gene therapy has expanded significantly since its inception in 1990. There is an everyday increase in clinical trials that focus on patients with threatening diseases, which have fewer remedial options.

Stem Cells:

There are non-specialized cells that renew constantly to produce more stem cells. They can mature, develop special function or change under specific growth conditions. Stem cells ultimately form all of the different types of cells that constitute the body. Stem cell research focuses on the potential of an undifferentiated stem cell, to produce a variety of other cells.

This therapy is at an experimental stage and it involves a laboratory process by which stem cells are grown and guided to a cell type by adding specific growth factors. These different cells are surgically implanted so that it can integrate into the diseased tissue, replace cells and reverse the effects of the disease.

Another process could be the implantation of undifferentiated stem cells and guide them to the differentiated cells in a patient's body. The objective is to replace damaged cells with healthy cells, and therefore it is called regenerative medicine. The optimistic view is that this process can be a renewable source of replacing cells and tissues to treat various diseases.

Nanotechnology:

Nanomedicine is the application of nanotechnology for improvement of human health. Basically, it is the manipulation of molecules and structures on a nanometer (one billion of a meter) or atomic scale.

Biotechnology nanomedicine harnesses living organism on a very limited scale. Nanoshells selectively target and destroy cancer cells at the cellular level. These shells are nanoscopic metallic lenses that act on specific organs, tissues, through the bloodstream. They have the capacity to capture infrared light, convert the same to heat, killing only the desired cancer cells.

Nanoparticles possess the shape of constructed carbon molecules, having the potential for drug delivery to target molecules or cells. They are also referred to as buckyballs and help to deliver drugs that do not dissolve in water. Because they are small in size, they have the potential to deliver most of the drug per volume. Scientific research on nanoparticles is being carried out to assess their capability to unclog blocked articles.

New Drug Delivery System:

Biomedical research is discovering new ways of drug delivery and its impact. One new development is that of microscopic particles called microsphere. They help to carry small quantities of drugs to their target through tiny holes that they possess. Structurally they resemble naturally occurring fats in cell membranes and spray mist into nose or mouth. Microsphere therapies are now being used for lung cancer and respiratory diseases. Constant research is being undertaken to utilize microspheres to deliver anticancer drugs to active tumors and for pain management.

Future Roadmap

Revolutionary advances in biotechnology research and innovation have benefitted millions of patients in the world. The cycle of discovering, developing and delivering novel medications to combat severe disease conditions is an ongoing process. Companies continue to pursue their efforts to address significant unmet needs. The future will surely unfold the fruits of biotechnology research in its quest to unveil newer remedies for combating the threat of disease in the world.

Biotech Startup Steps

The spirit of life science entrepreneurship and consequently formation of innovative hubs are flourishing throughout the world. It is difficult to reconcile to the fact that this industry is almost 50 years old. Significant changes have taken place since Herb Boyer, a professor at the University of California, San Francisco (UCSF) and Bob Swanson, a young entrepreneur and venture capitalist founded Genentech in 1976, which served as a stepping stone to the biotechnology industry. At that time these ventures involved only faculty members or biotechnology professionals. Today, the scenario has changed as graduate students or postdocs are venturing into these life science startups.

The Birth of a Startup

In 2009, Dan Widmaier was a graduate student at UCSF in synthetic biology. He researched on engineering Salmonella to produce and secrete spider silk. Spider silk protein is stronger than steel and tougher than body armor. But despite these qualities, the silk-extraction is a lengthy process and labor intensive and is used in only luxury textiles. But Dan saw this opportunity to streamline the extraction and production and convinced his lab mate Ethan Mirsky and David Breslauer of the University of California, Berkeley. Thus, Refactored Materials was born in 2009. They applied for small business grants from the National Foundation, and Department of Defense proposing to produce spider silk from engineered microbes for armor and medical device applications. They started a single bench incubator space at UCSF called QB3 Garage. They raised two venture rounds and targeted the textile market. In years to come expect a lot of innovation in athletic clothes which will be more breathable, socks to be softer and silk garments more durable, thanks to these grad students with a vision.

Turning Research into an Agent of Change

To have a meaningful impact on society drives scientists to discover and improve capabilities, better health standards and increase efficiency. Most of this work is done in universities where facilities are not always adequate, and thus a separate vehicle is necessary. This has been the primary factor since the inception of Genentech. Entrepreneurs need a separate industry as the conduit for translational applications.

Startups are the vehicle for this change for three key reasons. It can address key technical risks, decide on whether to embark or not on important decisions, and low capital with negligible overhead. It is advisable that startups should listen to their investors and advisors and act swiftly if they wish to survive. Every experiment must be based on a go / no-go option. Data must be publication worthy as millions of dollars are invested. Constant risk management and selection of the best market must be done, so as to explore several potential applications. Startups must have the ability to pivot, be nimble and ensure that the technology has a viable market and ensure financial returns for the founders. These young students and postdocs can dedicate time and energy which the academic faculty are not able to do. Therefore, science startups usually involve these graduate students who develop the original technology and thereby the sense of ownership becomes strong. They remain very passionate and motivated when their efforts bear fruit.

Advice Points

(QB3, the California Institute of Quantitative Biosciences have helped 200 startup teams. 65 have successfully raised funds within 18 months of approaching QB3. Two-thirds of these teams are postdocs or graduate students).

Identify the Unmet Need That Your Technology Addresses

One must clearly state the problem they are trying to solve. But the problem and its solution must have a large market in order to thrive. Niche markets are acceptable, but the source of capital will be fewer. Hence, development of a technology translating in high returns must be identified.

Build a High Quality, Well-Rounded Team

Startups are never created by an individual. Co-founders with matching skills have to be found. For instance, a cancer biologist has to tie up with a pharmacologist, or a person with clinical experience has to work with an engineer in order to manufacture the products. Therefore, having partners with different skillsets reaps multiple benefits, and thereby expands the company and gives confidence to the investors.

Faculty co-founders mostly remain as advisors and board members. But a team having young academics with a blend of individuals with startup experience, enhances credibility in front of investors. Hence, a well-rounded team is needed to focus on the company's vision and mission.

Understand Incentives, and Use Them to Drive Your Company to Success

Once a team is put in place, incentive programs must be initiated in order to get the best out of the team. Initially funding may be a constraint and therefore large salaries are ruled out. But offer of equity or shares will result in greater participation and help to produce high quality work. This will drive up the value of shares resulting in shareholders receiving better returns. In order to recruit the best available talent, equity plays a very significant role.

Get Quality Legal Advice

A good lawyer is an asset to a startup as all legal parameters have to be framed properly. Although good lawyers are expensive, many legal firms offer incentives for startups, often opting for deferred payments till funding is in place. It makes more sense to form a C-corporation if initially the advisors have to be offered equity. But if a startup is only limited to service, a Limited Liability Corporation is adequate. Online registration of companies may result in various future problems, so it is better to try to avoid it.

The most valuable asset is the intellectual property of the company and must be secured early. It has to be patented, the technology protected, and all terms of licensing made acceptable by the legal counsel.

Money, Money, Money – Search Under Every Rock

Sources of early-stage funding for startups like Small Business Innovation Research (SBIR), Science and Technology Translation Research (STTR), apart from federal grants and Venture Capital provide loans. Foundations, crowd funding, friends and family are also a source, so one has to explore all avenues. SBIRs and STTRs have an annual budget of $100 million. One-third of Startup in a Box graduates operated on SBIRs funding. National Institutes of Health, National Science Foundation, Department of Defense, and Department of Energy are also grant providers, and many successful ventures like Refactored Materials have benefited from these entities. Hence, leave no stone unturned, explore all possibilities. It is absolutely necessary to build trust with potential investors so that an affirmative nod is induced from them.

Respect Your Investors

Investor research is very important before a meeting in order to know their specific area of interest. This helps in explaining project details and application in specific areas for fund utilization. It is a myth that investors shy away from scientific ventures. The truth is that science investors try to understand the technology before they invest cash. Significant are the words of engineer and statistician William Edwards Deming, "In God we trust, all others must bring data."
Investors understand the market and its potential. It is better to listen to their advice even before they have invested. Their insight can help to identify opportunities and evolve strategic planning.

Be Unfocused at the Beginning, But Learn to Identify Opportunities

Platform technologies have multiple applications and diverse markets to pursue. Therefore, an easier path to revenue is preferable. Large markets maybe attractive but is fraught with regulation and risk. One has to explore an alternate route that can give better yield even if it is a niche market. The example of Refactored Materials not venturing in ballistic armor but taking on the textile industry is a case in point. One can always come back to other applications at the opportune time.

Identify Your White-Hot Risk and Use Your Time Wisely

There are many risks related to scientific technology market such as: technical / scientific risk, regulatory risk, and market risk. The greater the risk, the more difficult it is to obtain funding. So the entrepreneur has to gauge, understand and take time in evaluation of these risks. Only then he can focus on answering questions and decrease those risks in the eyes of the investor.

Test and Build Your Business Model – no, you do not need a business person – yes, you can use a scientific approach too

A very important facet of a startup is to understand its business model. This is based on how the company fits into the market, and its value proposition. Who are the customers and partners? How the product is relevant and so on. Thus, people will not be interested to use a diagnostic for an illness that has no current therapy. The best way to validate a business model is to talk directly to partners in a process developed by Steve Blank called "customer discovery". The founders are the most suitable people for this validation since they have a deep understanding of the technology and can make changes if needed. So as Blank says, "Get out of the building!" By this he means greater interaction with relevant people outside your comfort zone.

Be Lean

Money is the main factor in a startup. Therefore, preparation of a budget with emphasis on maximum utilization of resources on major activities must be maintained. It is not necessary to hire too many people. Rather it is better to engage someone who is willing to work as an advisor or interim CEO by offering equity in lieu of pay. Then the startup can focus on core skills and keep its operation on a low-key basis. Money can also be saved by outsourcing accounting work and pay by the hour or service. In other words, keep the operation lean and trim.

Tell a Story Without Giving Away Your Secrets

Only an idea does not make a company, execution and feedback from others are needed in order to approach investors and potential partners. The discussion must be non-confidential in nature without revealing all the facts of the project. Even while patenting intellectual property it would be wise to avoid describing all the details. This process will help to eliminate non-disclosure agreement (NDA) during initial meetings with potential partners. Venture capitals will never sign an NDA at the initial stage.

Inform Yourself

The key to success is to always stay informed. Constant interaction with entrepreneurs, technology experts and university alumni who have started their own ventures will result in the flow of more information. Even try to reach out to faculty who have founded companies and establish contact with those entrepreneurs who have succeeded in their projects.

Do Not Give Up, and Get Ready for the Best Roller Coaster Ride

Refactored Materials will help to revolutionize spider silk production for various applications on a large scale, and in an environment-friendly manner. Therefore, despite the many daunting problems faced, not a single entrepreneur has any misgivings in starting a company. As in academic science or in life, hurdles will always be present. But pursuing and achieving the goal will always be worth the effort. The classic example of this is the case of Refactored Materials.

www.ingramcontent.com/pod-product-compliance
Lightning Source LLC
Chambersburg PA
CBHW030542220526
45463CB00007B/2940